50 Recipes
Fast Metabolism Diet

Disclaimer and Terms of Use:

Effort has been made to ensure that the information in this book is accurate and complete, however, the author and the publisher do not warrant the accuracy of the information, text and graphics contained within the book due to the rapidly changing nature of science, research, known and unknown facts and internet. The Author and the publisher do not hold any responsibility for errors, omissions or contrary interpretation of the subject matter herein. This book is presented solely for motivational and informational purposes only.

Table of contents

Why should you consider following a fast metabolism diet?

If you gain weight faster than you can lose them or if you gain weight without eating too much it probably means that your have a slow metabolism. Unlike the lucky people who have a fast metabolism that allows them to eat what they want and when they want, the other ones need a change in the way they eat in order to accelerate their lazy metabolism. Fortunately, there is a special diet that can help you reactivate your metabolism.

Learn how to accelerate your metabolism by using this diet.

Find out what can you cook and what ingredients you can use!

50 Recipes For Fast Metabolism Diet

Tomatoes And Avocado Salad

Preparation time: 10 minutes
Servings: 4
Difficulty: easy

Ingredients:
3 tomatoes chopped
1 avocado sliced
1 red onion cubed
2 garlic cloves
50 ml olive oil
2 tablespoons lime juice
A pinch of salt.

Mix the tomatoes with the avocado.

Mix the lime juice with the olive oil, the salt and the crushed garlic.

Add the onion to the tomatoes and the avocado.

Add the salad dressing and serve it right away.

Zucchini And Marinated Veggies Salad

Preparation time: 15 minutes
Servings: 4
Difficulty: easy

Ingredients:
1 zucchini chopped
1 carrot chopped
1 bell pepper chopped
1 onion chopped
5 garlic cloves crushed
50 ml olive oil
2 tablespoons vinegar
1 teaspoon sugar
A pinch of salt and pepper

Mix the zucchini with the onion, the bell pepper and the carrot. Add the garlic to the salad.

Heat the oil in a pan at a medium temperature and add it to the salad.

Add the vinegar, the salt, the pepper and the sugar.

Mix everything very well.

Cover the salad and leave it in the fridge for 6-8 hours.

Cucumber And Mango Salad

Preparation time: 15 minutes
Servings: 2
Difficulty: easy

Ingredients:
1 mango sliced
250 grams cucumbers sliced
1 onion chopped
2 teaspoons olive oil
1 tablespoon lemon juice
A pinch of salt and pepper

Mix the mango with the cucumbers.

Add the onion.

Mix the lemon juice with salt and pepper and add it to the salad.

Add the olive oil; mix everything very well and enjoy!

Tomatoes, Corn And Olive Salad

Preparation time: 10 minutes
Servings: 2
Difficulty: easy

Ingredients:
3 tomatoes chopped
2 tablespoons canned corn
10 olives chopped
10 grams onion chopped
1 teaspoon olive oil
A pinch of salt

Mix the tomatoes with the corn, the olives and the onion.

Add the olive oil and the salt! Serve right away!

Tomatoes And Yogurt Salad

Preparation time: 15 minutes
Servings: 2
Difficulty: easy

Ingredients:
3 tomatoes sliced
1 bell pepper sliced
1 onion
100 grams yogurt
A pinch of salt

Mix the tomatoes with the bell pepper and the onion.

Add the yogurt and the salt.

Mix everything very well and serve right away.

Tabouleh Salad

Preparation time: 15 minutes
Servings: 4
Difficulty: easy

Ingredients:
4 bunches parsley chopped
3 tomatoes sliced
2 onions chopped
1 tablespoon fresh chopped mint
2 tablespoons bulgur soaked for 5 minutes
2 tablespoons pomegranate sauce
lemon juice
50 ml olive oil
A pinch of salt

Put the parsley in a salad bowl.

Add the onions to the parsley.

Add the tomatoes to the salad.

Add the bulgur.

Add the mint, the pomegranate sauce, the
lemon juice, the salt and the oil.

Peach And Bell Pepper Salad

Preparation time: 15 minutes
Servings: 4
Difficulty: easy

Ingredients:
3 peaches sliced
1 red bell pepper chopped
1 chili pepper chopped
1 red onion chopped
1 bunch parsley chopped
2 garlic cloves crushed
1 lemon
A pinch of salt

Put the peaches in a salad bowl.

Add the bell pepper and the chili pepper.

Add the onion, the garlic and the parsley.

Mix all the ingredients.

Add the juice from a lemon and the salt.

Serve right away.

Tuna Salad

Preparation time: 10 minutes
Servings: 4
Difficulty: easy

Ingredients:
300 grams salad mix (lettuce, spinach)
chopped
2 radishes
160 grams canned tuna
½ lemon juice
A pinch of salt and pepper

Put the salads in a salad bowl.

Add the canned tuna.

Add the lemon juice, salt and pepper and stir
everything very well.

Serve right away!

Italian Salad With Beetroot And Oranges

Preparation time: 30 minutes
Servings: 3
Difficulty: easy

Ingredients:
1 beetroot boiled and sliced
1 teaspoon balsamic vinegar
2 garlic cloves crushed
A handful of parsley chopped
½ cup orange juice
2 tablespoons olive oil
A pinch of salt and pepper

Mix the parsley with the garlic cloves and the beetroot.

Mix the vinegar with the olive oil and the orange juice.

Add this dressing to the salad.

Also add salt and pepper and serve right away.

Spring Salad

Preparation time: 15 minutes
Servings: 4
Difficulty: easy

Ingredients:
 500 grams fresh spinach chopped
1 lettuce chopped
1 radish chopped
1 onion chopped
1 teaspoon sugar
1 tablespoon olive oil
2 tablespoons vinegar
A pinch of oregano
200 grams tofu cheese
A pinch of salt

Put the spinach and the lettuce in a salad bowl.

Add the radish, the onion, the salt, the sugar,
the vinegar, the oregano and the oil.

Add the cheese, the olive oil and the salt.

Mix everything very well and serve right away.

Vinaigrette Salad

Preparation time: 60 minutes
Servings: 6
Difficulty: medium

Ingredients:
4 pink potatoes boiled and cubed
2 carrots boiled and chopped
2 beetroots boiled and cubed
1 onion chopped
5 pickled cucumbers chopped
50 ml olive oil
A pinch of salt and pepper

Mix the potatoes with the beetroot and the carrots.

Add the onion and the chopped cucumbers.

Add the oil, the salt and the pepper and serve right away.

Moroccan Fish With Veggies

Preparation time: 45 minutes
Servings: 4
Difficulty: easy

Ingredients:
1 pound fish fillets sliced
3 carrots cubed
3 bell peppers cubed
5 garlic cloves chopped
3 tomatoes chopped
3 tablespoons lemon juice
A pinch of salt
1 cup water
1 teaspoon sugar
50 ml olive oil
1 teaspoon grounded ginger
1 teaspoon sweet paprika
1 teaspoon turmeric
1 teaspoon grounded coriander
3 tablespoons chopped parsley

Mix the fish fillets with the lemon juice.

Use a large pot to arrange the veggies.

Put the bell peppers, the carrots and the garlic.

Add the fish, the sugar, the salt and the tomatoes.

Heat the oil in a frying pan at a medium temperature.

Add the spices and leave them to cook for 3 minutes.

Pour this mix over the veggies and over the fish.

Add a cup of water and leave everything to boil for 30 minutes.

Add the parsley and serve!

Eggplants And Beetroot Stew

Preparation time: 45 minutes
Servings: 4
Difficulty: easy

Ingredients:
500 grams eggplants cubed
300 grams beetroot chopped
1 onion chopped
2 tomatoes chopped
2 garlic cloves chopped
50 ml olive oil
A pinch salt

Heat the oil in a frying pan at a medium temperature and cook the onion for a few minutes.

Add the beetroot and leave it to cook for 15 minutes.

Add the tomatoes and leave them to cook for another 10 minutes.

Add the eggplants and stir.

Leave for another 10 minutes.

Add the garlic and the salt and leave for another 3 minutes.

Serve it hot or cold!

Green Beans With Garlic

Preparation time: 15 minutes
Servings: 2
Difficulty: easy

Ingredients:
500 grams green beans boiled for 10 minutes
2 onions chopped
½ cup water
1 tablespoon olive oil
2 garlic cloves
A pinch of salt

Heat a large frying pan at a high temperature with the olive oil and cook the onion.

Add the water and cook for another few minutes.

Add the green beans, stir everything and cook for another 5 minutes.

Add the garlic and some salt and serve right away.

Salmon Dish With Parsley Crust

Preparation time: 30 minutes
Servings: 4
Difficulty: easy

Ingredients:
500 grams salmon fillet
1 bunch parsley chopped
1 handful rosemary
 3 tablespoons olive oil
 A pinch of salt and pepper

 Put the fish in a tray.

Add the rosemary, salt, pepper and the olive oil.

Add the parsley.

Cover the tray with some tin foil and leave it in the oven at 339 F (180 C) for 30 minutes.

Serve right away.

Ginger And Avocado Soup

Preparation time: 15 minutes
Servings: 4
Difficulty: easy

Ingredients:
3 glasses of water
5 tablespoons olive oil
½ cup lemon juice
1 red bell pepper chopped
1 teaspoon of ginger
A pinch of salt
8 persimmons
100 grams celery chopped
1 handful of chopped parsley
200 grams radish
1 carrot chopped
200 grams cauliflower chopped
1 avocado chopped

Mix the water with the lemon juice, the salt, the ginger, the persimmons and the oil.

Blend everything with your blender.

Add the parsley, the celery and half of the bell pepper to the mix you prepared before.

Blend again for 5 minutes.

Pour this is a soup bowl.

Add the cauliflower and avocado.

Add the other half of the bell pepper, the carrot and the radish.

Add salt and serve right away.

Avocado And Sesame Cream Soup

Preparation time: 15 minutes
Servings: 2
Difficulty: easy

Ingredients:
1 avocado chopped
100 grams sesame seeds crushed
100 grams sunflower seeds crushed
1 tablespoon olive oil
A pinch of salt and pepper
200 ml water

Mix the avocado with the sesame seeds, the sunflower seeds and the olive oil in a blender.

Add salt and the water.

Mix until you obtain a cream.

Couscous With Olives

Preparation time: 15 minutes
Servings: 4
Difficulty: easy

Ingredients:
500 grams cauliflower
100 grams chopped olives
A handful of parsley chopped
½ cup lemon juice
50 ml olive oil
A pinch of salt and pepper
1 teaspoon curry powder (optional)

Blend the cauliflower very well until in your kitchen blended until it reaches the consistency of couscous.

Put the cauliflower couscous in a large bowl.

Add the parsley and the olives.

Add the lemon juice, the oil, salt, pepper and the curry powder. Enjoy!

Spinach And Garlic Stew

Preparation time: 30 minutes
Servings: 4
Difficulty: easy

Ingredients:
1 pound fresh spinach boiled for 2 minutes
1 onion chopped
½ cup of water
4 tablespoons tomatoes sauce
2 tablespoons sunflower oil
2 garlic cloves crushed
A pinch of salt

.

Heat a frying pan with the oil at a medium temperature and cook the onion.

Add half a cup of water and leave it to cook for 5 minutes.

Chop the spinach and add it to the onion.

Add the tomatoes sauce and stir everything.

Leave the stew to cook for 10 minutes.

Add the garlic and the salt at the end.

Serve while it's hot.

Ricotta, Zucchini And Ham Appetizer

Preparation time: 50 minutes
Servings: 4
Difficulty: easy

Ingredients:
200 grams flour
3 eggs
1 tablespoon olive oil
20 grams melted butter
2 tablespoons cream
4 tablespoons milk
A pinch of salt and pepper
130 grams fresh ricotta cheese
½ bunch chopped parsley
50 grams cubed ham
2 zucchinis sliced
1 teaspoon baking powder

Roll the zucchini slices.

Mix the eggs with the flour and the baking powder.

Add the butter, the cream, the milk, salt and pepper.

Add the ricotta, the parsley and the ham.

Mix very well.

Pour everything in a tray with 1 tablespoon of olive oil.

Add the zucchini rolls in the tray.

Cook in the preheated oven at 339 F (180 C) for 45 minutes

Rice And Veggie Salad

Preparation time: 15 minutes
Servings: 2
Difficulty: easy

Ingredients:
200 grams boiled rice
1 green bell pepper cubed
1 red bell pepper cubed
1 orange bell pepper cubed
2 tablespoons peas
1 carrot boiled
2 tablespoons green olives chopped
1 onion sliced
2 tablespoons olive oil
A pinch of salt
½ bunch parsley chopped

Mix the bell peppers with the olives, the onion and the parsley.

Add the carrot, the peas and the rice.

Add the salt and the olive oil.

Mix very well and serve right away!

Tuna, Corn And Green Beans Salad

Preparation time: 15 minutes
Servings: 4
Difficulty: easy

Ingredients:
1 can of tuna
2 boiled and cubed potatoes
1 onion chopped
1 boiled egg sliced
5 cherry tomatoes cubed
50 grams green beans
50 grams corn
50 grams olives chopped
A pinch of dill chopped
5 leaves rucolla
5 leaves lettuce
2 tablespoons olive oil
2 tablespoons lemon juice
A pinch of salt and pepper
1 teaspoon mustard

Mix the potatoes, the corn, the lettuce and the green beans.

Add the olives, the onion, the dill, the tuna and the tomatoes.

Mix the lemon juice with the salt, the pepper, the mustard and the olive oil.

Add the salad dressing over the salad and mix everything.

Serve right away.

Carrots, Caraway And Mustard Salad

Preparation time: 15 minutes
Servings: 4
Difficulty: easy

Ingredients:
1 pound carrots sliced and boiled
½ caraway
1 lemon
 A pinch of salt and pepper
2 tablespoons mustard
2 tablespoons melted butter

Mix the carrots with the caraway, the melted butter.

Add the salt, the pepper, the mustard and the butter.

Add the lemon juice at the end and serve right away!

Spinach And Garlic Dish

Preparation time: 15 minutes
Servings: 4
Difficulty: easy

Ingredients:
1 pound fresh spinach chopped
2 tablespoons olive oil
7 crushed garlic cloves
A pinch of salt and pepper
1 tablespoon butter
½ cup lemon juice

Heat the olive oil at a medium temperature in a frying pan and cook the garlic for about 1 minute.

Add the spinach, the salt and the pepper.

Leave everything to boil for 2 minutes.

Add the lemon juice and serve while it's hot!

Russian Carrots Salad

Preparation time: 10 minutes
Servings: 6
Difficulty: easy

Ingredients:
1 pound carrots grated
4 garlic cloves crushed
1 medium onion chopped
2 tablespoons coriander seeds
4 tablespoons olive oil
3 tablespoons vinegar
½ bunch parsley chopped
A pinch of salt, pepper and sweet paprika
1 tablespoons honey
2 teaspoons sugar

Heat at a medium temperature 1 tablespoons of oil and cook the onion for 5 minutes.

Mix the carrots with the garlic, the coriander seeds and 3 tablespoons of oil.

Add the vinegar, the parsley, the sugar, the honey, the salt and the pepper.

Add the paprika and the onion at the end.

Serve after 4 hours.

Asparagus Vinaigrette

Preparation time: 10 minutes
Servings: 4
Difficulty: easy

Ingredients:
800 grams fresh asparagus
1/3 cup balsamic vinegar
2 tablespoons water
2 tablespoons olive oil
2 tablespoons mustard
2 tablespoons chopped parsley
2 teaspoons chopped tarragon
1 tablespoon chopped onion

Cut the asparagus and boil it for 5 minutes.

Put it in cold water.

Mix the olive oil with the balsamic vinegar, the water and the mustard.

Add the parsley, the tarragon and the onion.

Add the asparagus and serve right away.

Apples And Cabbage Salad

Preparation time: 10 minutes
Servings: 6
Difficulty: easy

Ingredients:
½ red cabbage chopped
½ white cabbage chopped
½ grated carrot
2 green apples sliced
3 tablespoons raisins
2 teaspoons lemon juice
3 teaspoons apple vinegar
½ cup yogurt
2 tablespoon olive oil
A pinch of salt and pepper

Mix the cabbages with the apples and add the lemon juice as well.

Add the carrots and the raisins.

Mix the yogurt with the vinegar, the oil, salt and pepper.

Mix the salad with the dressing and serve after 30 minutes.

Simple Salad

Preparation time: 10 minutes
Servings: 6
Difficulty: easy

Ingredients:
2 small oranges sliced
1 lemon (juiced)
½ red onion chopped
2 tablespoons olive oil
½ crushed nuts
10 olives sliced
5 handfuls lettuce and spinach chopped

Heat a frying pan with 1 tablespoon of olive oil at a medium temperature and cook the nuts for 5 minutes.

Mix the onion with the lemon juice and 2 tablespoons olive oil.

Add the salt and the pepper.

Put the lettuce and the spinach in a salad bowl.

Add the oranges, the nuts and the onion.

Potatoes And Radish Salad

Preparation time: 10 minutes
Servings: 6
Difficulty: easy

Ingredients:
1 pound potatoes boiled and cubed
12 radishes chopped
1 handful chopped spinach
½ cup chopped onion
½ cucumbers chopped
3 tablespoons olive oil
3 tablespoons vinegar
A pinch of salt and pepper

Mix the potatoes with the olive oil.

Add the onion and the radishes.

Add the spinach, the cucumber, the salt, the pepper and the vinegar.

Serve right away.

Carrots And Raisins Salad

Preparation time: 10 minutes
Servings: 4
Difficulty: easy

Ingredients:
3 cups of grated carrots
2 big apples sliced
¼ cup raisins
½ cup cooking cream
3 tablespoons olive oil
½ cup lemon juice
1 teaspoon sugar
¼ teaspoon cinnamon
¼ teaspoon nutmeg
1/8 teaspoon allspice

Sprinkle the lemon juice on the apple slices.

Mix them with the carrots, the raisins, salt and pepper.

Add the cinnamon, the nutmeg and the allspice.

Mix the cooking cream with the sugar and add to the salad.

Add the lemon juice and mix everything.

Serve right away.

Eggplant Salad

Preparation time: 15 minutes
Servings: 4
Difficulty: easy

Ingredients:
1 big eggplant grilled and peeled
1 onion chopped
1 zucchini boiled
½ cup lemon juice
1 tablespoon chopped parsley
1 tablespoon olive oil
1 crushed garlic clove
A pinch of salt

Use your kitchen blended to blend the eggplant.

Add the zucchini and the oil and blend for another 3 minutes.

Add the onion and the garlic and blend for another 2 minutes.

Add the lemon juice, the salt and the parsley and blend for another 3 minutes.

Serve after it gets cold.

Tomatoes And Mint Salad

Preparation time: 10 minutes
Servings: 4
Difficulty: easy

Ingredients:
6 tomatoes sliced
1 small onion chopped
1 tablespoon fresh mint chopped
1 lemon
1 tablespoon fresh coriander chopped
A pinch of salt

Mix the onion with the mint, the coriander and the tomatoes.

Add the lemon juice and the salt.

Leave in the fridge for half an hour and then serve.

Watermelon Salad With Feta Cheese

Preparation time: 15 minutes
Servings: 4
Difficulty: easy

Ingredients:
2 slices of watermelon cubed
1 cup feta cheese cubed
½ red onion chopped
1 tablespoon fresh mint chopped

Mix the watermelon with the feta cheese and the red onion.

Add the mint.

Serve right away!

Gazpacho

Preparation time: 15 minutes
Servings: 4
Difficulty: easy

Ingredients:
¼ pound tomatoes chopped
½ onions chopped
1 small cucumber chopped
1 green bell pepper sliced
A pinch of salt
2 tablespoons olive oil
2 tablespoons vinegar
2 garlic cloves crushed
Bread croutons

Mix the tomatoes with the onion.

Add the garlic, the vinegar and the salt.

Put everything in a blender and mix everything.

Add the olive oil and mix again.

Serve in small bowls with bread croutons.

Tomatoes And Garlic Soup

Preparation time: 15 minutes
Servings: 4
Difficulty: easy

Ingredients:
4 garlic cloves crushed
50 ml olive oil
1 liter tomatoes juice
1 teaspoon salt
1 teaspoon brown sugar
1 handful fresh basil chopped

Heat up a frying pan at a medium temperature with 10 ml of olive oil.

Cook the garlic for 3-4 minutes.

Heat up another pan with 40 ml oil at a medium temperature.

Add the tomatoes juice and stir for a few minutes.

Add the garlic and leave the soup to boil for 7 minutes.

Add the salt, the sugar and the mint.

Serve when it gets cold.

Carrots And Oranges Soup

Preparation time: 20 minutes
Servings: 4
Difficulty: easy

Ingredients:
1 liter vegetables stock
4 carrots chopped
3 potatoes chopped
Juice from 1 orange
4 tablespoons cooking cream
1 bunch parsley chopped
A pinch of salt and pepper

Boil the chicken stock.

Add the carrots and the potatoes.

Leave everything to boil for 20 minutes.

Take out the veggies and put them in a kitchen blender.

Add the orange juice and blend for a few minutes.

Add the stock and mix again.

Add the parsley and the cream at the end.

Add the salt and the pepper and enjoy!

Fresh Cheese Cream With Dill

Preparation time: 5 minutes
Servings: 4
Difficulty: easy

Ingredients:
500 grams fresh cheese crushed
300 grams cooking cream
1 bunch chopped dill

Mix the cheese with the cream and the dill.

Leave everything in the fridge for about 1 hour.

Enjoy!

Baked Veggies

Preparation time: 20 minutes
Servings: 4
Difficulty: easy

Ingredients:
3 potatoes cubed
1 zucchini cubed
1 carrot cubed
1 bell pepper sliced
1 celery root cubed
1 onion sliced
50 ml olive oil
1 cup of hot water
A pinch of salt

Put all the veggies in a tray.

Add the olive oil, the salt and the hot water.

Introduce the tray in the oven at 338 F (170 C) for 20 minutes.

Serve right away.

Mexican Fish Soup

Preparation time: 20 minutes
Servings: 6
Difficulty: easy

Ingredients:
5 cups water
½ cup white wine
3 chopped onions
2 garlic cloves crushed
1 hot chili pepper sliced
2 zucchinis cubed
2 tomatoes peeled and sliced
450 grams fish fillets
2 tablespoons vinegar
3 tablespoons olive oil
1 cup fresh chopped coriander
A pinch of salt

Mix the water with the white wine, the onions, the garlic and the hot pepper.

Leave them to boil for 10 minutes.

Add the zucchinis and the tomatoes.

After 5 minutes add the fish fillets and leave everything to boil for another 10 minutes.

Add the vinegar, the olive oil, the coriander and the salt.

Serve right away!

Oregano And Zucchini Dish

Preparation time: 10 minutes
Servings: 4
Difficulty: easy

Ingredients:
650 grams zucchini boiled and cubed
1 teaspoon oregano
1 teaspoon melted butter
A pinch of salt and pepper

Mix the zucchini with the oregano and the melted butter.

Add salt and pepper and serve right away!

Spicy Salmon Fillet

Preparation time: 20 minutes
Servings: 4
Difficulty: easy

Ingredients:
600 grams salmon fillets sliced
1 bunch fresh tarragon chopped
1 bunch parsley chopped
1 lemon sliced
½ bunch dill chopped
2 tablespoons olive oil
100 ml vegetable stock
1 tablespoon capers
1 teaspoon mustard
2 teaspoon Tabasco sauce
1 onion chopped
A pinch of salt and pepper

Heat up a frying pan with 1 tablespoon of olive oil at a medium temperature and cook the lemon slices.

Add the fish and cook for 5 minutes.

Add the onion and cook for another 2 minutes.

Mix the tarragon with the parsley and the dill in a blender.

Add 1 tablespoon olive oil, the vegetable soup.

Add the capers, the mustard and the Tabasco sauce and mix.

Place the salmon fillets on plates. Add the mix you prepared earlier.

Add salt and pepper and serve right away.

Nisa Salad

Preparation time: 15 minutes
Servings: 4
Difficulty: easy

Ingredients:
1 lettuce chopped
1 radish chopped
1 red bell pepper sliced
5 tomatoes sliced
1 tuna can
1 red onion chopped
4 boiled eggs sliced
2 garlic cloves crushed
50 grams olives sliced
4 tablespoons olive oil
2 tablespoons vinegar
A pinch of salt and pepper

Mix the lettuce with the bell peppers, the radish, the tomatoes and the eggs.

Add the tuna, the onion, the olives and the garlic.

Add salt, pepper, the vinegar and the oil at the end.

Serve right away.

Spicy Soup

Preparation time: 15 minutes
Servings: 4
Difficulty: easy

Ingredients:
2 onions chopped
2 garlic cloves chopped
1 tablespoon olive oil
300 grams boiled green beans
425 grams boiled beans
2 tomatoes
2 tablespoons grated parmesan
1 teaspoon fresh chopped basil
A pinch of salt and pepper

Heat up a large pot with the olive oil at a medium temperature and cook the onion and the garlic for 3 minutes.

Add the green beans, the beans and water to cover the veggies.

Boil for 10 minutes.

Add the tomatoes, the parmesan, salt and pepper.

Add the basil at the end and serve right away!

Cabbage Soup

Preparation time: 20 minutes
Servings: 4
Difficulty: easy

Ingredients:
1 celery root chopped
1 medium cabbage chopped
4 carrots chopped
6 tomatoes chopped
2 red bell peppers chopped
1 bunch parsley chopped
2 bay leaves
4 garlic cloves crushed
A pinch of salt and pepper
1 teaspoon of rosemary chopped
1 teaspoon tarragon chopped
 500 ml water

Mix the water with the tomatoes.

Boil this mix for 5 minutes.

Add the onion, the cabbage, the celery, the carrots, the bell peppers, the salt and pepper.

Leave everything to boil for 10 minutes.

Add the bay leaves and the garlic.

Then, add the tarragon, the rosemary.

Serve hot or cold!

Garlic Soup

Preparation time: 15 minutes
Servings: 4
Difficulty: easy

Ingredients:
15 garlic cloves crushed
2 teaspoons olive oil
1 onion chopped
1 liter veggies stock
50 grams grated parmesan
100 grams cooking cream
½ cup lemon juice
A pinch of salt and pepper
1 handful chopped parsley
100 grams croutons

Heat up a pot with the olive oil at a medium temperature.

Cook the onion and the garlic for 4 minutes.

Add the veggies stock and boil for 6 minutes.

Add the cooking cream and boil everything for another 5 minutes.

Add the salt, the pepper and the parsley at the end.

Serve the soup hot with the croutons.

Apple and potatoes soup

Preparation time: 20 minutes
Servings: 4
Difficulty: easy

Ingredients:
1 teaspoon olive oil
1 medium onion chopped
1 apple sliced
1 teaspoon crushed garlic
½ cup white wine
5 potatoes cubed
A pinch of salt and pepper
1 cup apple cider or apple juice
¾ cup non fat milk
3 cups water
2 teaspoons grated parmesan
½ teaspoon nutmeg

Heat up a frying pan with the olive oil at a medium temperature and cook the onion, the apple and the garlic.

Cook for 5-6 minutes.

Add the wine and cook for another 4 minutes.

Add the potatoes, the salt and the water and boil for 15 minutes.

Add the milk, the apple cider, the parmesan, the nutmeg, salt and pepper.

Boil for another 5 minutes.

Serve right away.

Chinese Soup

Preparation time: 35 minutes
Servings: 4
Difficulty: easy

Ingredients:
300 grams chicken breast
500 ml water
2 garlic cloves crushed
1 tablespoon grated ginger
2 tablespoons soy sauce
2 onions chopped
100 grams mushrooms sliced
50 grams soup noodles
100 grams cabbage chopped
3 coriander leaves chopped
1 chili pepper chopped
A pinch of salt and pepper

Boil the chicken breast in water for 15 minutes.

Add the onion, the garlic, the cabbage, the mushrooms and the ginger.

Boil for another 10 minutes.

Add the soy sauce, the chili pepper and the noodles.

Cook for another 5 minutes.

Add the coriander, salt and pepper.

Serve right away!

Fennel Soup

Preparation time: 35 minutes
Servings: 4
Difficulty: easy

Ingredients:
2 tablespoons olive oil
300 ml water
1 onion chopped
1 bell pepper chopped
2 carrots chopped
½ celery root chopped
3 fennels sliced
2 garlic cloves crushed
2 tablespoons nuts crushed
A pinch of saffron, salt and pepper

Boil the vegetables in water for 15 minutes.

Add the fennel and the garlic.

Boil for another 10 minutes.

Use your kitchen blender to blend the soup when it's done.

Add the saffron, the olive oil, the salt, the pepper and the nuts.

Serve right away!

Veggie Pudding

Preparation time: 35 minutes
Servings: 4
Difficulty: easy

Ingredients:
150 grams carrots chopped
150 grams potatoes chopped
150 grams apples sliced
1 teaspoon nutmeg
200 grams sugar
A pinch of salt
1 teaspoon baking powder
150 grams raisins
1 teaspoon mineral water
1 teaspoon cinnamon
1 egg white
2 teaspoons olive oil

Mix all the veggies and the apple with the nutmeg, the sugar, the salt, the baking power, the mineral water and the cinnamon.

Add the egg white, the olive oil and the raisins.

Put everything in a tray and introduce in the oven for 1 hour at about 212 F (100 C).

Serve while it's still warm.

Caponata

Preparation time: 60 minutes
Servings: 6
Difficulty: easy

Ingredients:
900 grams eggplant chopped
230 grams celery chopped
60 ml olive oil
80 grams onion chopped
2 tablespoons vinegar
5 tomatoes chopped
2 tablespoons tomatoes juice
2 tablespoons pine seeds
A pinch of salt and pepper

Heat up a frying pan with the olive oil at a medium temperature and cook the eggplants for 10 minutes.

Add the celery and the onion and cook for another 6 minutes.

Add the vinegar, the tomatoes, the tomatoes juice, the salt and the pepper.

Cook for another 15 minutes.

Add the pine seeds and serve right away!

Conclusion

Don't hesitate to try all the recipes presented because they will help you boost up your metabolism. If you try these dishes you will see how your health will improve in no time. Your appearance will change as well and you will impress everyone around you! The metabolism diet is easy to follow and you should definitely try it!

www.ingramcontent.com/pod-product-compliance
Lightning Source LLC
Chambersburg PA
CBHW070325290526
45791CB00003B/1256